CROHN'S DISEASE DIET COOKBOOK

Delicious And Easy Recipes For Managing Symptoms, Reducing Inflammation, And Promoting Gut Health

DR ELIAN GRIFFIN

Copyright © [Elian Griffin] [2024]. All rights reserved.

Without the publisher's prior written consent, no portion of this publication may be copied, distributed, or transmitted in any way, including by photocopying, recording, or other mechanical or electronic means, with the exception of brief quotations used in all critical reviews.

DISCLAIMER

The nutritional recommendations and recipes in this book are meant solely for informative reasons. They are not meant to replace the counsel, diagnosis, or care of a qualified medical expert. If you have any doubts about a medical condition or dietary requirements, you should always see your physician or another trained healthcare expert.

All reasonable efforts have been taken by the author and publisher to ensure that the information contained in this book is correct as of the date of publication. Recommendations may alter, though, as medical knowledge is always changing. When using any of the recipes or instructions found here, the user assumes all liability and assumes no risk, whether personal or otherwise. People who have certain dietary requirements or medical issues should speak with a healthcare provider for personalized guidance. The given recipes are only ideas; you may need to adjust them to suit your own nutritional needs, tastes, and tolerances.

When you use this book, you agree to release the publisher, the author, and their representatives from any liability for any claims, damages, liabilities, costs, or expenditures resulting from your use of the book.

TABLE OF CONTENTS

CHAPTER ONE 13
CROHN'S DISEASE DIET INTRODUCTION 13
KNOWING ABOUT CROHN'S DISEASE AND HOW NUTRITION AFFECTS IT 13
THE ROLE THAT NUTRITION PLAYS IN SYMPTOM MANAGEMENT 14
HOW USING THIS COOKBOOK CAN RAISE ONE'S STANDARD OF LIVING 15
ADVICE ON HOW TO MAKE THE MOST OF THE COOKBOOK 16
A SUMMARY OF THE TYPICAL INGREDIENTS USED IN THE RECIPES .. 17

CHAPTER TWO 19
OVERVIEW OF DIET AND CROHN'S DISEASE 19
THE FUNDAMENTALS OF CROHN'S DISEASE AND HOW IT AFFECTS DIGESTION 19
DIET IS IMPORTANT FOR MANAGING SYMPTOMS 20
THE IMPORTANCE OF A BALANCED DIET FOR GENERAL HEALTH 21
RECOGNIZING INTOLERANCES AND FOOD TRIGGERS 22
AN OVERVIEW OF THE CROHN'S DISEASE-FRIENDLY DIET 23

CHAPTER THREE 25
ORGANIZING YOUR KITCHEN 25
ESSENTIAL COOKING UTENSILS AND KITCHENWARE 25
HOW TO STOCK YOUR PANTRY FOR A CROHN'S DISEASE-FRIENDLY DIET 26
SELECTING HIGH-QUALITY SUBSTANCES FOR YOUR RECIPES 27
RECOGNIZING FOOD LABELS AND INGREDIENTS TO STEER CLEAR 28
EASY COOKING RECIPES FOR QUICK AND EASY MEAL 30

- CHAPTER FOUR 31
  - MEALS PLANNING AND PREPARATION 31
    - REQUIREMENTS FOR CROHN'S DISEASE MEAL PLANNING 31
    - TECHNIQUES FOR BATCH COOKING TO SAVE TIME AND 32
    - ADVICE FOR GROCERY PURCHASING WHILE CONSIDERING A CROHN'S-FRIENDLY DIET 33
    - MEAL PLANNING IN ADVANCE FOR BUSY DAYS OR FLARE-UPS 34
    - MAKING A MEAL PLAN THAT IS FLEXIBLE ENOUGH TO MEET 35
  - BREAKFAST RECIPES 36
    - HEALTHY AND SIMPLE-TO-COMB BREAKFAST IDEAS 36
    - SMOOTHIE RECIPES FOR AN EASY AND SATISFYING MORNING 37
    - PORRIDGES & BOWLS FOR BREAKFAST PACKED WITH VITAL 39
    - INNOVATIVE METHODS FOR INCLUDING PROTEIN AND FIBER IN 40
    - ADVICE FOR ORGANIZING YOUR SCHEDULE AND PREPARING 42
  - RECIPES FOR LUNCH AND DINNER 44
    - SOPHISTICATED SOUPS AND STEWS WITH MINIMAL STOMACH IMPACT 44
    - EASY AND QUICK ONE-POT LUNCH OR DINNER RECIPES 45
    - SALADS THAT ARE WELL-BALANCED AND CONTAIN CROHN'S-FRIENDLY 46
    - RECIPES FOR MAIN COURSES WITH LEAN PROTEINS AND 47
    - SOME IDEAS FOR ADAPTING CLASSIC RECIPES TO A CROHN'S 48
  - SIDES AND SNACKS 49
    - HEALTHY SNACK IDEAS TO REDUCE CRAVINGS WITHOUT MAKING SYMPTOMS WORSE 49
    - HANDMADE SPREADS AND DIPS TO GO WITH VEGGIES OR 50

- SIDE DISHES PACKED WITH NUTRIENTS TO GO WITH MAIN.............51
- CONVENIENT SNACKS TO EAT ON THE GO..52
- ADVICE ON PORTION CONTROL AND MINDFUL SNACKING...............53
- DRINKS AND SMOOTHIES..54
  - RECIPES FOR HYDRATING DRINKS TO PROMOTE DIGESTIVE HEALTH54
  - COMBINATIONS OF SMOOTHIES TO INCREASE YOUR VITAMIN.........55
  - HERBAL INFUSIONS AND TEAS TO CALM THE DIGESTIVE 57
  - ADVICE ON HOW TO DRINK ENOUGH WATER DURING THE..............58
  - INNOVATIVE METHODS FOR ADDING NUTRITIOUS SUPPLEMENTS ..59
- SWEETS AND TREATS 62
  - DESSERT RECIPES THAT ARE FREE OF GUILT AND USE CROHN'S FRIENDLY SUBSTANCES 62
  - SWEETS MADE OF FRUIT FOR A NATURAL SUGAR FIX........................63
  - DELICIOUS CANDIES PREPARED WITH NUTRITIOUS TWISTS..............64
  - ADVICE FOR EATING DESSERTS MODERATELY AND WITHOUT..........65
  - DESSERT SUBSTITUTES THAT FULFILL CRAVINGS WITHOUT 66
- CHAPTER FIVE..69
  - PARTICULAR DIETS AND LIMITATIONS 69
    - ADVICE FOR MEETING PARTICULAR NUTRITIONAL REQUIREMENTS.69
    - RECIPES FIT FOR A VEGETARIAN OR VEGAN DIET 70
    - LOW-RESIDUE FOOD SELECTIONS FOR PERIODS OF OUTBURSTS.......71
    - ADDING ANTI-INFLAMMATORY SUBSTANCES TO YOUR FOODS........72
    - ADAPTING RECIPES TO INDIVIDUAL DIETARY RESTRICTIONS AND 74
- CHAPTER SIX...75
  - FAQS & FREQUENTLY ASKED QUESTIONS 75

HANDLING VARIATIONS IN WEIGHT WITH A CROHN'S DIET............... 75
MANAGING NUTRITIONAL LIMITATIONS IN SOCIAL CONTEXTS 76
TAKING CARE OF THE COMMON NUTRIENT DEFICIENCIES IN 78
SUGGESTIONS FOR EATING OUT WHILE FOLLOWING A CROHN'S..... 79
RECOGNIZING SUPPLEMENTS' FUNCTION IN SYMPTOM................... 80

ABOUT THE BOOK

Understanding food triggers and intolerances is crucial, as it provides readers with insights into creating a diet that supports digestive health and overall well-being. The comprehensive guide "Crohn's Disease Diet Cookbook" is an invaluable resource for individuals navigating the complexities of managing Crohn's disease through nutrition. It begins by exploring the fundamentals of Crohn's disease, shedding light on its impact on digestion and emphasizing the crucial role of diet in symptom management.

The cookbook's ability to improve the quality of life for people with Crohn's disease is at the heart of its significance. It provides a wide range of recipes that are formulated to be easy on the stomach while still being high in vital nutrients, enabling people to enjoy tasty meals without aggravating their symptoms. The cookbook's useful tips for efficient use guarantee that it is accessible and easy to use, advising users on everything from setting up the kitchen and choosing ingredients to basic cooking methods that make meal preparation easier.

To support digestive health, the cookbook's structured approach starts with foundational knowledge and eases readers into meal planning strategies that accommodate busy schedules and fluctuations in health. Breakfast options prioritize nutrition and ease of digestion, such as smoothies and nutrient-packed porridges. Comforting yet nutritious lunch and dinner recipes include soups, stews, and protein-rich main courses.

Ideas for snacks and side dishes offer nutritious substitutes that satisfy cravings without going against diet restrictions; drink recipes emphasize hydration and support for the digestive system with nutrient-rich smoothies and herbal infusions; desserts offer decadence with careful ingredient selections that guarantee sweetness without causing discomfort; and the cookbook also covers dietary specialties like vegan or gluten-free diets, offering flexibility and inclusivity in meal planning.

The cookbook covers a wide range of issues and frequently asked questions, including how to deal with weight fluctuations, how to handle dietary restrictions in social situations, and how to address nutrient deficiencies that are common in Crohn's patients. It also explores the role of supplements in symptom management, providing a comprehensive approach to dietary support.

The "Crohn's Disease Diet Cookbook" is essentially more than just a recipe book; it's a customized manual that encourages people to make educated dietary decisions and take control of their health, leading to a balanced and pleasurable eating style while coping with the difficulties brought on by Crohn's disease.

CHAPTER ONE

CROHN'S DISEASE DIET INTRODUCTION

KNOWING ABOUT CROHN'S DISEASE AND HOW NUTRITION AFFECTS IT

The management of Crohn's disease involves understanding how certain foods can trigger or exacerbate symptoms due to inflammation. Since the disease varies in severity and location within the digestive system, individualized dietary adjustments are crucial for symptom management. For example, some people may find relief by avoiding high-fiber foods that can aggravate inflammation, while others may need to avoid dairy or gluten.

Crohn's disease is a chronic inflammatory condition that primarily affects the gastrointestinal tract, causing symptoms like abdominal pain, diarrhea, fatigue, and weight loss.

Knowing the complexities of Crohn's disease allows one to customize diets to reduce symptoms and aid in healing. By recognizing trigger foods and taking an anti-inflammatory stance, people can better control flare-ups and improve their general health. This cookbook makes it easier to find appropriate meals that are easy on the stomach but high in vital nutrients.

THE ROLE THAT NUTRITION PLAYS IN SYMPTOM MANAGEMENT

A well-balanced diet can help alleviate symptoms, support healing, and improve overall well-being. For example, including foods rich in antioxidants, omega-3 fatty acids, and probiotics can help reduce inflammation and support gut health.

On the other hand, processed foods, high in sugar, and saturated fats may exacerbate symptoms and trigger flare-ups. Nutrition is crucial in managing Crohn's disease because it directly impacts inflammation levels and digestive health.

Nutrition is important for more than just managing symptoms; it also boosts immunity, increases energy, and generally improves quality of life. This cookbook focuses on simple, high-nutrient recipes that are easy to digest, so people with Crohn's disease can still enjoy tasty meals without sacrificing their health objectives.

HOW USING THIS COOKBOOK CAN RAISE ONE'S STANDARD OF LIVING

With a variety of simple meal ideas, this cookbook aims to reduce the anxiety and stress that come with meal planning for people who are managing a chronic illness. All of the recipes are made with the health and well-being of Crohn's Disease patients in mind, with an emphasis on the digestive system and optimal nutrition. This allows people to maintain a balanced diet without compromising taste or enjoyment.

Beyond just recipes, the cookbook provides helpful advice and insights into meal planning, ingredient selection, and dietary modifications unique to Crohn's disease. By encouraging a healthy relationship with food and streamlining the process of preparing nourishing meals, this resource seeks to improve the overall quality of life for people coping with Crohn's disease.

ADVICE ON HOW TO MAKE THE MOST OF THE COOKBOOK

To get the most out of this cookbook, read through the introductory sections first, as they contain dietary principles specific to Crohn's Disease. Next, consider meal prepping ahead of time to save time and make sure you always have nutrient-dense options on hand. Finally, try out a variety of recipes until you find ones that work best for your particular triggers and preferences.

You can effectively manage Crohn's Disease and enhance your overall well-being by incorporating these tips into your culinary routine. Make use of the ingredient lists and nutritional information provided for each recipe to help you make informed decisions that support your health goals. Don't hesitate to modify recipes based on personal preferences or dietary restrictions.

Keep a journal to track how different foods affect your symptoms over time so that you can improve your meal plans.

A SUMMARY OF THE TYPICAL INGREDIENTS USED IN THE RECIPES

Numerous nutrient-dense ingredients, such as lean proteins (like chicken, fish, and tofu) that supply essential amino acids without overwhelming the digestive system, and fresh fruits and vegetables (like leafy greens, berries, and squash) that provide vitamins, minerals, and fiber to support gut health and overall well-being are common ingredients found in this cookbook's recipes.

Healthy fats from sources like olive oil, avocados, and nuts provide essential fatty acids that have anti-inflammatory properties and contribute to heart health; herbs, spices, and low-acidic sauces add flavor without compromising digestive comfort.

CHAPTER TWO

OVERVIEW OF DIET AND CROHN'S DISEASE

THE FUNDAMENTALS OF CROHN'S DISEASE AND HOW IT AFFECTS DIGESTION

While it can occur anywhere from the mouth to the anus, Crohn's disease primarily affects the gastrointestinal tract, causing inflammation and damage to the lining of the digestive system. It primarily affects the ileum, which is the end of the small intestine, and the colon, which is the beginning of the large intestine. Although symptoms can vary greatly from person to person, they often include abdominal pain, diarrhea, fatigue, weight loss, and malnutrition due to impaired nutrient absorption.

Crohn's disease is characterized by inflammation that impairs the normal function of the digestive system and can result in complications like fistulas, strictures, and abscesses. The disease is difficult to manage because it often alternates between active flare-ups and periods of remission, necessitating ongoing monitoring and treatment adjustments.

Knowing how Crohn's disease affects digestion is essential for controlling symptoms and enhancing quality of life. People can make educated dietary decisions to reduce pain and promote overall health by understanding how inflammation impacts nutrient absorption and gastrointestinal function.

DIET IS IMPORTANT FOR MANAGING SYMPTOMS

A well-planned diet helps reduce inflammation, promotes healing of the intestinal lining, and supports the body's immune system. It is important to note that diet alone cannot cure Crohn's disease, but it can greatly influence the frequency and severity of flare-ups.

Certain foods have the potential to exacerbate symptoms or worsen inflammation in people with Crohn's disease. It is important to recognize and stay away from foods that cause inflammation, such as foods high in fat or spice, dairy products, gluten, and some raw fruits and vegetables. It is also important to stay properly hydrated and make sure you are getting enough vitamins and minerals in your diet.

Consulting with a physician or a registered dietitian with expertise in gastrointestinal disorders can offer individualized advice on developing a diet plan that suits personal requirements and preferences.

THE IMPORTANCE OF A BALANCED DIET FOR GENERAL HEALTH

Everybody benefits from a well-balanced diet, but those with Crohn's disease benefit even more from it. A diet rich in a range of nutrient-dense foods promotes healing, immune system support, and overall health while also helping to manage symptoms by lowering inflammation.

Lean proteins (fish, poultry, and tofu) supply essential amino acids for immune system support and tissue repair; complex carbohydrates (whole grains and starchy vegetables) that provide sustained energy; and fiber (fiber helps maintain regular digestion and a healthy gut microbiome) are important parts of a well-balanced diet for people with Crohn's disease.

Fruits and vegetables, when well tolerated, provide essential vitamins, minerals, and antioxidants that support immune function and overall wellness. By emphasizing nutrient-dense foods and minimizing processed foods and sugars, people can optimize their diet to support both digestive health and overall well-being. Healthy fats from sources like olive oil, nuts, and seeds can help reduce inflammation and support heart health.

RECOGNIZING INTOLERANCES AND FOOD TRIGGERS

The treatment of Crohn's disease symptoms is greatly influenced by the identification and elimination of food triggers and intolerances. Common trigger foods include dairy products, gluten-containing grains, high-fat foods, spicy foods, and foods high in fiber. Certain foods can also increase inflammation or cause gastrointestinal discomfort, which can lead to increased symptoms and possible flare-ups.

Keeping a thorough food journal and recording any symptoms that arise after consuming particular foods are important steps in identifying individual food triggers. Dietitians and healthcare professionals can assist in identifying troublesome foods and creating a personalized diet plan that reduces discomfort and aids in symptom management.

Managing food intolerances through dietary modifications, such as choosing lactose-free dairy products or gluten-free grains, can alleviate digestive distress and support overall gut health.

AN OVERVIEW OF THE CROHN'S DISEASE-FRIENDLY DIET

Foods that are high in fiber, difficult to digest, or known triggers for inflammation are often limited or avoided. A Crohn's-friendly diet focuses on reducing inflammation, promoting healing, and minimizing gastrointestinal discomfort. It typically includes easily digestible foods that are gentle on the digestive system, such as cooked fruits and vegetables, lean proteins, and refined grains.

Nutrient-dense foods, including those rich in vitamins, minerals, and antioxidants, are prioritized to support immune function and overall health. The diet emphasizes hydration and encourages adequate fluid intake to support digestion and prevent dehydration, which is especially important during periods of flare-ups when diarrhea and fluid loss may be more pronounced.

By fostering a healthy balance of gut bacteria, probiotics-rich foods like yogurt with live cultures or fermented vegetables may also be helpful for some people. However, individual tolerance to probiotics should be monitored, as some individuals with Crohn's disease may find that certain probiotics strains worsen their symptoms.

Implementing a Crohn's-friendly diet entails tailoring food selections to each person's tolerance, symptoms, and nutritional requirements.

CHAPTER THREE

ORGANIZING YOUR KITCHEN

ESSENTIAL COOKING UTENSILS AND KITCHENWARE

Having the proper tools and equipment is the first step in preparing a kitchen to support a Crohn's disease-friendly diet. Investing in a good quality chef's knife, paring knife, and serrated knife will allow for precise cutting and chopping, reducing the effort required to prepare ingredients. A sturdy cutting board, preferably made of wood or plastic, will also protect your countertops and ensure a clean surface for food preparation.

A slow cooker or pressure cooker can be a lifesaver for preparing tender, easily digested meals with little effort; these appliances are great for making soups, stews, and casseroles that can be cooked slowly to break down fibrous foods. Various sizes of pots and pans are another essential set of tools. Notably, non-stick pans require less oil, making cooking healthier and cleanup easier.

A food processor or blender is a great tool for pureeing vegetables and creating smoothies, which can be easier on the digestive system. Other important kitchen tools include measuring cups and spoons, a digital kitchen scale, and a decent set of mixing bowls. Precise measurement is crucial for preserving the consistency and safety of your Crohn's-friendly recipes.

HOW TO STOCK YOUR PANTRY FOR A CROHN'S DISEASE-FRIENDLY DIET

Incorporating a Crohn's-friendly diet into your pantry organization can greatly expedite your cooking process and guarantee that you always have the necessary ingredients on hand. Begin by classifying items like grains, canned goods, spices, and snacks. Store items like rice, quinoa, and gluten-free flours in airtight containers so that you can see what you have at a glance and they stay fresh.

The next step is to label everything. You can label containers with a label maker or just masking tape and a marker. Labeling your pantry helps you find what you need quickly. You can also use expiration dates on these labels to make sure you use ingredients while they're still fresh. By keeping a running inventory of pantry staples, you can avoid running out of important items.

Use baskets or bins to group similar items, such as breakfast foods or baking supplies. This method of organization not only makes meal prep easier but also reduces the stress of finding ingredients, allowing you to focus on preparing nutritious meals that are gentle on your digestive system.

SELECTING HIGH-QUALITY SUBSTANCES FOR YOUR RECIPES

To create wholesome, Crohn's-friendly meals, start with high-quality ingredients: look for seasonal produce at local farmers' markets, as these are often fresher and more nutrient-dense; incorporate a variety of colors and types of vegetables in your diet to ensure a broad range of vitamins and minerals; and source fresh fruits and vegetables, preferably organic, to avoid pesticides that can irritate the gut.

When it comes to protein, choose lean meats such as turkey, chicken, and fish. These are usually easier to digest than red meats and offer essential amino acids without being overly fat. As for plant-based proteins, think about tofu, tempeh, and thoroughly cooked legumes that have been reduced in fiber. Eggs are another great source of protein that is easy to digest and can be prepared in a variety of ways.

Read labels to avoid added sugars and preservatives that could trigger symptoms. When it comes to dairy, choose lactose-free options or plant-based milks like almond or oat milk.

RECOGNIZING FOOD LABELS AND INGREDIENTS TO STEER CLEAR OF

To manage a Crohn's-friendly diet, you must read food labels. Packaged foods have their ingredients listed in descending order of weight, meaning that the first few ingredients make up the majority of the product. Look for products with short, easily recognizable ingredient lists and steer clear of those with lengthy lists of chemicals or preservatives.

A lot of packaged foods, especially processed ones, contain hidden sources of potential irritants like gluten, dairy, and high-fiber ingredients. Gluten is commonly found in sauces, soups, and processed meats; dairy may turn up in unexpected places like baked goods and snacks; and for some people, high-fiber ingredients like whole grains and specific vegetables can exacerbate symptoms.

Knowing what is contained in food labels can help you make informed decisions that support your overall health and digestive health. For example, look for foods low in sodium and added sugars, as these can cause inflammation and digestive discomfort. Be wary of terms like "natural flavors" and "spices," as they can sometimes mask unwanted additives.

EASY COOKING RECIPES FOR QUICK AND EASY MEAL PREPARATION

Cooking can be made less intimidating and more fun by simplifying methods such as steaming, which is a gentle way to cook vegetables while retaining nutrients; it works best for leafy greens, carrots, and squash. Just place the vegetables in a steamer basket over boiling water, cover, and cook until tender.

Baking, also known as roasting, is another fantastic method that works well with meats, fish, and root vegetables. Simply preheat your oven, season your ingredients with a little olive oil and herbs, and bake until cooked through. Roasting brings out the flavors of the food naturally and is a great hands-off method for batch cooking, which allows you to cook multiple meals at once and save time and effort throughout the week.

Using a non-stick pan or wok can help reduce the need for excess oil. For quick and simple meals, try stir-frying, which is cooking small pieces of food quickly over high heat with a small amount of oil.

CHAPTER FOUR

MEALS PLANNING AND PREPARATION

REQUIREMENTS FOR CROHN'S DISEASE MEAL PLANNING

Crohn's disease meal planning requires careful consideration of dietary restrictions and individual health needs. Make a list of foods and ingredients that you can tolerate based on your unique triggers and nutritional needs.

Aim for a balanced diet that includes foods that are easy to digest, like cooked vegetables, lean proteins, and low-fiber grains. Plan meals that are easy on the digestive system to reduce discomfort and flare-ups.

Plan with simplicity and variety in mind. Choose foods that are simple to make and digest, like soups, steamed veggies, and well-cooked grains. Divide meals into small, frequent servings throughout the day to sustain energy levels and aid indigestion. Watch portion sizes to prevent overindulging, which can worsen symptoms.

To customize your meal plan and guarantee adequate nutrition, speak with a dietitian who specializes in Crohn's disease.

TECHNIQUES FOR BATCH COOKING TO SAVE TIME AND ENERGY

A useful tactic for handling Crohn's disease meals is batch cooking, which lets you make bigger amounts of food ahead of time and freeze it for later use. Recipes like stews, casseroles, and pasta dishes work well for freezing and reheating. Cooked meals can be divided into individual servings for easy access on hectic days or during flare-ups.

Set aside a specific time each week to prepare meals; label and date meals before putting them in the fridge or freezer to track freshness and rotation; and adjust portion sizes based on your appetite and nutritional needs to ensure balanced meals and prevent waste. Efficient cooking techniques, such as pressure cooking or slow cooking, can save time and energy while ensuring food safety and quality.

ADVICE FOR GROCERY PURCHASING WHILE CONSIDERING A CROHN'S-FRIENDLY DIET

When grocery shopping, people with Crohn's disease must be extremely mindful of their dietary needs and food triggers. To start, make a list of the foods you want to buy based on your meal plan and favorite foods. Try to stick to whole, fresh foods like lean proteins, soft fruits, and well-cooked vegetables. Low-fiber items like white rice, pasta, and peeled fruits will help reduce gastrointestinal distress.

Shop at off-peak hours to avoid crowds and stress, which can affect digestion and general well-being. Look into online grocery options for added convenience and accessibility, especially during times of low energy or flare-ups.

Read food labels carefully to avoid additives, preservatives, and ingredients that may aggravate symptoms. Choose organic or locally sourced produce when possible to reduce exposure to pesticides and chemicals.

MEAL PLANNING IN ADVANCE FOR BUSY DAYS OR FLARE-UPS

Meal prep containers can be used to portion out servings for easy access throughout the week. Versatile ingredients that can be readily adapted to suit changing dietary needs and preferences. Planning is key to managing Crohn's Disease during busy days or flare-ups. Soups, casseroles, and salads are good examples of recipes that are easy to batch-cook and store.

To ensure consistency and reduce stress at the last minute, set aside a specific time each week for meal preparation. To maximize meal enjoyment and satisfaction, use efficient cooking techniques such as roasting, steaming, or sautéing to preserve nutrients and enhance digestibility.

Label and date prepared meals before storing them in the refrigerator or freezer to maintain freshness and minimize food waste.

MAKING A MEAL PLAN THAT IS FLEXIBLE ENOUGH TO MEET YOUR HEALTH NEEDS

A flexible meal plan is essential for managing Crohn's disease because it enables you to adjust to shifting requirements and symptoms. To prevent flare-ups, start by identifying foods and intolerances that trigger symptoms. Then, include a range of nutrient-dense foods, such as cooked vegetables, lean proteins, and low-residue grains, to promote general health and well-being.

Prioritize moderation and balance when creating your meal plan. Choose foods that are simple to digest and kind to the digestive tract, like smoothies, soups, and well-cooked meats. Try new flavors and cooking techniques to make meals engaging and fun. Keep an eye on portion sizes and meal frequency to sustain energy levels and aid in the digestive system. Consult a dietitian or healthcare provider with expertise in Crohn's disease to personalize your meal plan and guarantee adequate nutrition.

BREAKFAST RECIPES

HEALTHY AND SIMPLE-TO-COMB BREAKFAST IDEAS

For those who are managing Crohn's disease, it's important to find nourishing and easily digestible breakfast ideas. For example, you can start your morning with scrambled eggs with well-cooked vegetables, which will provide you with protein and vitamins without putting too much strain on your digestive system. Alternatively, you can have yogurt topped with ripe bananas and a sprinkle of ground flaxseeds for extra fiber and probiotics. Both of these options are nourishing and easy on your stomach, so you can start your day feeling good.

Smoothies are a great way to start your day when you need a quick and nutritious breakfast. Blend easily digestible fruits like ripe bananas, papaya, and strawberries with lactose-free yogurt or almond milk. You can also add a tablespoon of chia seeds or nut butter to boost protein and healthy fats for sustained energy levels.

Smoothies are quick to make and can be customized to suit your taste preferences and nutritional needs.

Breakfast bowls and porridges are a great option for something heartier. If you're feeling particularly indulgent, try a warm rice porridge with low-FODMAP vegetables and a poached egg for extra protein.

You can also customize these bowls with different toppings like nuts, seeds, or a drizzle of olive oil. Either way, you'll be eating a filling, nutrient-dense meal that will help your digestive system.

SMOOTHIE RECIPES FOR AN EASY AND SATISFYING MORNING

Smoothies are a great way to start the day when you're looking for easy-to-digest foods. To start, make a simple green smoothie with spinach, cucumber, and a ripe pear blended with coconut water. This combination will give you plenty of hydration as well as important vitamins and minerals without overwhelming your digestive system.

If you want to add more protein, you can also add a scoop of plain whey protein or plant-based protein powder.

A tropical smoothie made with coconut milk or water, pineapple, mango, and ginger is another cooling choice. The ginger helps with digestion and gives the smoothie a tangy kick, and the fruits naturally provide sweetness and vital nutrients. You can also add a tablespoon of ground flaxseeds or hemp seeds for extra fiber and omega-3 fatty acids, which support gut health and reduce inflammation.

Smoothies can be tailored to your taste preferences and dietary needs by adding natural sweeteners like honey or dates to adjust the sweetness level. For a decadent and creamy twist, try a chocolate banana smoothie made with unsweetened cocoa powder, ripe bananas, and almond butter blended with almond milk. This combination offers a balance of carbohydrates, healthy fats, and protein, making it a satisfying breakfast or snack option.

PORRIDGES & BOWLS FOR BREAKFAST PACKED WITH VITAL NUTRIENTS

Start with a savory oatmeal bowl topped with sautéed spinach, a poached egg, and a sprinkle of nutritional yeast for extra B vitamins. This combination provides fiber, protein, and vitamins essential for maintaining energy levels throughout the morning while supporting gut health. Breakfast bowls and porridges are versatile options packed with essential nutrients, ideal for those managing Crohn's disease.

Instead, try making a quinoa breakfast bowl with cooked quinoa combined with diced cucumbers, cherry tomatoes, and olive oil. You can also add some fresh herbs, like cilantro or parsley, for flavor and antioxidants.

Quinoa is gluten-free and easily digested, so it's a good option for people with sensitive stomachs. You can also personalize your bowls by adding avocado slices, pumpkin seeds, or a squeeze of lemon juice for extra freshness and nutrition.

Warm rice porridge, made with brown rice cooked in low-sodium chicken broth or vegetable broth, is a comforting option. This hearty dish is gentle on the stomach yet satisfying, ensuring you start your day with a nutritious meal that supports digestive comfort and overall well-being. Top the porridge with steamed carrots, peas, and shredded chicken or tofu for protein. Season with turmeric, ginger, and a dash of sea salt for added flavor and anti-inflammatory properties.

INNOVATIVE METHODS FOR INCLUDING PROTEIN AND FIBER IN BREAKFAST MEALS

For people with Crohn's disease, breakfast meals must include both fiber and protein to maintain digestive health and effectively manage symptoms. To start your day off right, make a high-fiber smoothie bowl with blended mixed berries, spinach, and a scoop of hemp protein powder. Top the bowl with granola, chia seeds, and a dollop of Greek yogurt for extra protein and probiotics. This will guarantee a nutritious and well-balanced breakfast.

Try this savory veggie frittata with ingredients like bell peppers, spinach, and zucchini. Vegetables provide vitamins and minerals that are important for overall health, and eggs are a high-quality source of protein. Bake the frittata in the oven until it sets and turns golden brown, then slice it into portions for convenient grab-and-go breakfasts all week. Serve with a side of mixed greens or a slice of gluten-free toast for a complete meal.

Another inventive concept is a quinoa breakfast salad, which consists of cooked quinoa combined with diced avocado, cherry tomatoes, and edamame beans. It is dressed with a homemade lemon-tahini dressing for extra taste and creaminess. Edamame and quinoa are good plant-based protein sources, and avocado offers fiber and healthy fats. This salad can be made ahead of time and refrigerated, making it a healthy and easy breakfast choice.

ADVICE FOR ORGANIZING YOUR SCHEDULE AND PREPARING BREAKFAST IN BULK

A weekly meal plan that includes a variety of breakfast options, like smoothie packs, frittatas, and overnight oats, can make meal preparation easier and ensure you have nourishing options on hand—especially when managing Crohn's disease. Make sure your recipe selections are simple to make in bulk and can be kept in the freezer or refrigerator for easy access on busy mornings.

Think about making a big batch of overnight oats using rolled oats, chia seeds, almond milk, and your preferred sweeteners or fruits. Once the oats are divided among individual mason jars or containers, chill them in the refrigerator overnight. The next morning, just open a jar, top with your preferred toppings (like almonds or fresh berries), and have a healthy, satisfying breakfast.

Another idea for batch cooking is to make mini vegetable and cheese frittatas in a muffin tin. Beat eggs, grated cheese, and diced vegetables like onions, bell peppers, and spinach. Pour the mixture into muffin cups that have been greased and bake until set. Once cooled, store the frittatas in an airtight container in the freezer or refrigerator. Warm them up in the oven or microwave for a quick and healthy breakfast option that you can enjoy all week long.

Finally, put together smoothie packs by dividing your preferred smoothie components—such as protein powders, frozen fruits, and leafy greens—into separate freezer bags. Freeze the packs for up to a month. When you're ready to eat, just empty the contents of a pack into a blender, add your preferred liquid, and process until smooth. This efficient way guarantees that you can have a nutrient-dense smoothie ready in a matter of minutes, making it a great option for busy mornings or days when you need a quick and well-balanced breakfast option.

RECIPES FOR LUNCH AND DINNER

SOPHISTICATED SOUPS AND STEWS WITH MINIMAL STOMACH IMPACT

Soups and stews are calming and simple to digest when dealing with Crohn's disease. Choose homemade or low-sodium broths to limit consumption.

Begin with vegetables such as carrots, celery, and potatoes, which are easy on the stomach and full of nutrients; add lean proteins like chicken or tofu for extra protein without overwhelming the digestive system; season lightly with herbs like parsley or dill, which can add flavor without irritating the stomach.

To prepare, chop veggies finely to help with digestion and to make sure they cook through. Simmer over low heat to blend flavors and soften textures, which is easier on sensitive digestive systems. Use a small amount of olive oil or coconut milk for richness instead of heavy cream, which can aggravate symptoms. Serve soups and stews warm, not hot, to avoid discomfort.

These recipes are not only nourishing, but they also aid in effectively managing symptoms.

EASY AND QUICK ONE-POT LUNCH OR DINNER RECIPES

For people with Crohn's disease, one-pot meals are the best option because they reduce mess and streamline the cooking process. Start with easily digested ingredients, like quinoa, brown rice, or gluten-free pasta; add vegetables, like zucchini, spinach, or bell peppers, for vitamins and fiber; add lean proteins, like turkey, fish, or lentils, for extra nutrition without upsetting the digestive system; and season with herbs and spices instead of thick sauces to bring out the flavor while keeping the dish light on the stomach.

These meals can be tailored to individual preferences and dietary requirements, offering a well-rounded and fulfilling option for lunch or dinner. To prepare, begin by lightly sautéing vegetables in olive oil or broth to soften them. Add grains or pasta along with liquid (broth or water) and bring to a gentle simmer. Cook until grains are tender and flavors have melded together.

Be careful not to overcook to maintain the nutritional integrity of ingredients.

SALADS THAT ARE WELL-BALANCED AND CONTAIN CROHN'S-FRIENDLY

When prepared with consideration, salads can be both nutrient-dense and easy on the digestive tract. Begin with a base of easily digestible, high-vitamin leafy greens, such as kale or spinach; add cooked vegetables, such as roasted sweet potatoes or steamed broccoli, for texture and fiber; add protein sources, such as grilled chicken, tofu, or boiled eggs, to make the salad more filling and well-balanced; and use a light dressing, such as olive oil, lemon juice, and herbs, to steer clear of heavy fats and artificial additives.

To assemble, cut ingredients into small pieces for easier chewing and digestion. Toss gently with the dressing right before serving to preserve flavor and freshness. Steer clear of raw onions, garlic, or spicy ingredients as these can aggravate symptoms. These salads are adaptable and can be made with seasonal fruits and vegetables, which makes them a healthy and energizing option for a Crohn's disease diet.

RECIPES FOR MAIN COURSES WITH LEAN PROTEINS AND NUTRIENT-DENSE SIDES

To support overall health and manage the symptoms of Crohn's disease, main courses should center around lean proteins and nutrient-dense sides. Lean proteins, such as grilled chicken, turkey, or fish, are rich in essential amino acids and easy to digest. For fiber, vitamins, and minerals, pair with sides like steamed vegetables, quinoa pilaf, or mashed sweet potatoes. Season with mild herbs and spices to add flavor without overpowering the digestive system.

To preserve the nutritional value and digestibility of proteins, they should be cooked, grilled, or baked with minimal added fats. Vegetables should be steamed or lightly sautéed to preserve their texture and nutrients. Whole grains, such as buckwheat or brown rice, should be included to provide sustained energy without causing discomfort to the digestive tract.

These recipes are meant to be well-balanced and filling, supporting a diet that is Crohn's disease-friendly while guaranteeing sufficient nutrition and mouthwatering flavors.

SOME IDEAS FOR ADAPTING CLASSIC RECIPES TO A CROHN'S DIET

The key to adjusting to a Crohn's diet and still enjoying favorite recipes is to modify them. You can start by cutting back on or swapping out high-fat ingredients for healthier ones, like avocado or olive oil; replace dairy with lactose-free alternatives or plant-based alternatives, like almond milk or coconut yogurt; and reduce your intake of gluten, which can exacerbate symptoms, by using gluten-free flours or grains, like rice or quinoa, in place of wheat products.

Increase the amount of herbs, spices, and citrus juices to enhance flavor without adding too much salt or sugar; try baking, steaming, or grilling to preserve nutrients and enhance digestibility.

SIDES AND SNACKS

HEALTHY SNACK IDEAS TO REDUCE CRAVINGS WITHOUT MAKING SYMPTOMS WORSE

It can be difficult for people with Crohn's disease to find satisfying snacks that are also easy on the stomach. Try low-fiber, easily digested snacks like rice cakes with almond butter or Greek yogurt with honey and a sprinkle of nuts; these will give you a good balance of protein and carbohydrates without overwhelming your digestive system. Another excellent option is a smoothie made with easily digested fruits, like bananas or mangoes, blended with lactose-free yogurt or almond milk for creaminess.

Savory options include homemade vegetable soups or broths, which are cooked until the vegetables are soft and easily digested. These can be prepared in large quantities and frozen for easy on-the-go snacks during the week. When selecting snacks, look for foods that are easy on the stomach and steer clear of triggers like high-fat or spicy foods.

This helps to balance the nutritional requirements of Crohn's disease with craving management.

HANDMADE SPREADS AND DIPS TO GO WITH VEGGIES OR CRACKERS

Making your spreads and dips gives you complete control over what's in them and can be customized to fit your specific dietary needs. For example, a basic hummus consisting of chickpeas, tahini, lemon juice, and olive oil is a great way to get some protein and healthy fats and goes well with cucumber slices or gluten-free crackers. Another option is a yogurt-based dip flavored with herbs like mint or dill, which can be combined with grated cucumber or carrots for extra texture and nutrients.

If you would rather something sweeter, consider preparing a fruit salsa with diced mango, pineapple, and strawberries, along with some lime juice and chopped mint. This light salsa goes well with gluten-free tortilla chips or as a grilled chicken or fish topping. When you make your dips and spreads, you can stay away from the preservatives and additives that are frequently found in store-bought varieties, making your snack healthier and better for your digestive system.

SIDE DISHES PACKED WITH NUTRIENTS TO GO WITH MAIN COURSES

Aside from improving the color and fiber content of any plate, adding nutrient-dense side dishes like roasted carrots, zucchini, and bell peppers tossed with olive oil and seasoned with herbs like thyme or rosemary can also improve flavor and nutritional value without sacrificing digestive health. Quinoa or couscous salads topped with cherry tomatoes, chopped herbs, and a light vinaigrette are another delicious way to combine protein and carbohydrates.

More substantial options include mashed sweet potatoes seasoned with a little nutmeg or cinnamon. Sweet potatoes are high in vitamins and minerals and easily digested when cooked through. Alternatively, nutrient-dense side dishes like steamed or sautéed greens like spinach or kale go well with lean proteins like grilled chicken or fish. By concentrating on digestibility and nutrient density, you can make side dishes that not only meet your nutritional needs but also make your meals more enjoyable.

CONVENIENT SNACKS TO EAT ON THE GO

When managing Crohn's disease, you need to be able to manage your busy schedule with portable snacks that are light on the stomach. For example, you can make your granola bars with oats, seeds, and a little honey for sweetness. These bars offer a healthy balance of carbohydrates and protein, which is perfect for keeping your energy levels up all day. Another easy option is a trail mix, which is a combination of nuts, dried fruits, and dark chocolate chips for a satisfying blend of flavors and textures.

For a quick and wholesome snack, pack individual portions of lactose-free yogurt or cottage cheese with fresh berries or a small serving of gluten-free crackers. If you'd rather have something savory, pack individual portions of rice cakes with avocado slices and a dash of sea salt. These snacks are simple to make and convenient to eat on the go, so you can continue to eat a balanced diet even while managing your symptoms.

ADVICE ON PORTION CONTROL AND MINDFUL SNACKING

Maintaining overall digestive health and controlling Crohn's disease symptoms require mindful snacking. To begin, observe hunger cues and select snacks that satiate cravings without taxing the digestive system. Portion control is crucial, so choose smaller, more frequent snacks throughout the day instead of larger meals that may be more difficult to digest. Store healthful snacks in easily accessible snack-sized containers or bags.

You can better manage your Crohn's disease symptoms by practicing mindful snacking and portion control. You can also enjoy a variety of nourishing and satisfying snacks throughout the day. Avoid distractions when snacking to fully enjoy and appreciate the flavors and textures of your food.

DRINKS AND SMOOTHIES

RECIPES FOR HYDRATING DRINKS TO PROMOTE DIGESTIVE HEALTH

Here are some refreshing drink recipes that support digestive wellness in addition to hydrating. For starters, try making cucumber mint-infused water by slicing fresh cucumbers and adding them to a pitcher of water along with a handful of mint leaves. Then, let the mixture sit in the refrigerator for a few hours so the flavors can meld. This drink not only hydrates but also has a calming effect on the digestive tract because of the cooling properties of cucumber and the digestive benefits of mint.

Equal parts coconut water and aloe vera juice make a refreshing drink that supports hydration and digestive health. You can squeeze in some lemon juice for extra flavor and vitamin C. Coconut water is naturally hydrating and rich in electrolytes, which can be beneficial during flare-ups.

Aloe vera juice is known for its anti-inflammatory properties and can help soothe the digestive lining.

Ginger tea is a warm option that can help with digestion and reduce inflammation. To make ginger tea, grate fresh ginger root into a pot of boiling water, let it simmer for about 10 minutes, then strain the liquid into a cup. You can add a little honey or lemon if you like. Ginger tea is a great option for people with Crohn's disease because it helps with digestion and keeps the digestive tract comfortable.

COMBINATIONS OF SMOOTHIES TO INCREASE YOUR VITAMIN AND MINERAL COUNT

While managing Crohn's disease, smoothies are a convenient way to pack in nutrients. Here are some delicious combinations to try that will give you a boost of essential vitamins and minerals. Start with a classic green smoothie: blend fresh spinach or kale with a banana, almond milk, and a spoonful of almond butter. The vitamins A, C, and K found in green leafy vegetables are important for immune function and general health. The banana adds creaminess and potassium, which can help replenish electrolytes lost during digestive problems.

A berry antioxidant smoothie is another delicious option. Blend a small amount of Greek yogurt, coconut water, and a handful of mixed berries, such as strawberries, blueberries, and raspberries. Greek yogurt adds probiotics, which are good bacteria that support gut health, and berries are full of antioxidants that can help reduce inflammation in the digestive tract. Enjoy this colorful smoothie as a nutrient-rich snack or as a meal replacement.

A refreshing smoothie that provides a range of nutrients to support digestive comfort and overall wellness can be made with fresh pineapple chunks, grated ginger, coconut milk, and a handful of spinach. Pineapple contains bromelain, an enzyme that aids in digestion and reduces inflammation. Ginger adds a zesty kick and helps settle the stomach. Coconut milk provides healthy fats and a creamy texture.

HERBAL INFUSIONS AND TEAS TO CALM THE DIGESTIVE SYSTEM

Herbal teas and infusions can provide relief to people suffering from Crohn's disease. One popular option is peppermint tea, which helps to ease bloating by relaxing the muscles in the digestive tract. To make peppermint tea, steep dried or fresh peppermint leaves in hot water for 5 to 10 minutes, strain, and drink. If you would like, you can add a little honey for sweetness.

Another mild option that can help reduce inflammation and encourage relaxation is chamomile tea (steep chamomile flowers in hot water for several minutes, then strain and sip slowly). It is well-known for its anti-inflammatory qualities and can be especially calming during Crohn's disease flare-ups. Additionally, because it is caffeine-free, it can be consumed any time of day or right before bed to help encourage sound sleep.

To make turmeric tea, add a pinch of black pepper to enhance the absorption of curcumin. Simmer grated fresh turmeric root or powdered turmeric in hot water for about 10 minutes. This golden-hued tea supports digestive health and makes a warming, comforting beverage option for those who prefer a slightly spicy option. Turmeric contains curcumin, a compound with potent anti-inflammatory and antioxidant properties.

ADVICE ON HOW TO DRINK ENOUGH WATER DURING THE DAY

Here are some doable strategies to make sure you stay hydrated throughout the day: drink a glass of water in the morning that has been infused with slices of cucumber or lemon. This easy step can jump-start hydration and give you a refreshing boost of vitamins and minerals. Keep a reusable water bottle with you throughout the day to keep track of your water intake and make staying hydrated convenient.

Include foods that are high in water in your diet, such as citrus fruits like watermelon and oranges, as well as vegetables like cucumbers and celery. These foods will not only help you meet your daily fluid needs, but they will also supply vital nutrients that will support the health of your digestive system. If you are the type of person who often forgets to drink water, set a reminder on your phone or use an app. Flavored waters and herbal teas can be tasty substitutes for regular water and will help you drink more fluids overall.

Prioritize hydration during Crohn's disease flare-ups by drinking electrolyte-rich liquids (like coconut water or diluted sports drinks) to replace lost fluids and minerals; stay away from excessive caffeine and alcohol as these can also lead to dehydration. You can support the health of your digestive system and your general well-being by choosing foods and beverages that are high in water content.

INNOVATIVE METHODS FOR ADDING NUTRITIOUS SUPPLEMENTS TO DRINKS

Here are some creative ways to incorporate nutritional supplements into your beverages. Protein is important for immune system function and tissue repair, so it's especially important for people with Crohn's disease who may have increased nutrient needs.

Start with a protein-packed smoothie by adding a scoop of high-quality protein powder to your favorite smoothie recipe. Nutritional supplements can help manage Crohn's disease by providing essential nutrients and supporting overall health.

Adding a probiotics to your daily routine can help support digestive comfort and help maintain a healthy balance of gut bacteria; look for a probiotics supplement that is specifically formulated for people with digestive issues and pay close attention to the dosage instructions. Powdered greens supplements can also be added to smoothies or juices to increase your intake of vitamins, minerals, and antioxidants.

You can boost your nutritional intake and support your overall health goals by incorporating supplements into delicious and nutritious beverages.

If you need extra help absorbing vitamins and minerals, try blending a liquid multivitamin supplement into a fruit or vegetable juice. Liquid forms of vitamins are often easier to digest and absorb, making them a convenient option for people with Crohn's disease who may have nutrient absorption challenges. Make sure you speak with your healthcare provider before starting any new supplements to ensure they are appropriate for your specific needs and condition.

SWEETS AND TREATS

DESSERT RECIPES THAT ARE FREE OF GUILT AND USE CROHN'S FRIENDLY SUBSTANCES

Choosing low-fiber fruits like bananas and applesauce, which can be used to make tasty and easy-to-digest treats, is a good way to create guilt-free desserts for people with Crohn's disease.

For example, ripe bananas, almond flour, and a little honey can be combined to make banana bread, which is not only a moist, sweet dessert but also a nutritious treat that is packed with essential nutrients without irritating the digestive system.

Yogurt can also give your dessert recipes a creamy texture without being too heavy on the stomach. Lactose-free yogurt can help those who are lactose intolerant, which is a common problem for Crohn's patients. These parfaits are easy to make ahead of time and keep in the refrigerator, making them a convenient and healthful dessert option.

Layers of smooth, pureed fruits topped with a drizzle of honey offer a refreshing and light option.

Nut butter cookies, which are made with a mixture of nut butter, eggs, and a small amount of sugar, are a soft and satisfying treat that is high in protein and healthy fats, offering a nourishing option without taxing the digestive system. Another great option is to use smooth nut butter, like almond or peanut butter, in your recipes.

SWEETS MADE OF FRUIT FOR A NATURAL SUGAR FIX

Smoothies prepared with ripe bananas, seedless watermelon, and a splash of lactose-free milk can create a refreshing and nutrient-rich drink; a little honey or a dash of cinnamon can enhance the flavor without using refined sugars, making it an excellent dessert or snack option. Fruit-based sweets can be a fantastic way to get a natural sugar fix while keeping Crohn's symptoms at bay.

The result is a warm, comforting dessert that is naturally sweet and easy on the stomach.

Pairing baked apples with a dollop of lactose-free yogurt or a sprinkle of nutmeg can add an extra layer of flavor. Baked fruits can also be a delicious and easy-to-digest dessert. For example, core an apple and fill it with a mixture of honey, cinnamon, and a small amount of finely chopped nuts before baking until tender.

Fruit sorbets are a great substitute for traditional ice cream because they are naturally sweet and satisfying for those with Crohn's disease. Fruit sorbets are made from pureed, frozen fruits such as mangoes, blueberries, and strawberries. Blending the fruits until smooth and then freezing them results in a creamy texture without the need for added sugars or dairy.

DELICIOUS CANDIES PREPARED WITH NUTRITIOUS TWISTS

For example, chocolate avocado mousse combines the rich taste of chocolate with the creamy texture of avocados; simply blend ripe avocados with cocoa powder and a touch of honey until smooth. Packed with healthy fats and antioxidants, this dessert is both indulgent and nutritious. People with Crohn's disease don't have to give up on their favorite treats because they can enjoy them guilt-free.

Another example is making thick and creamy pudding with chia seeds, almond milk, and a little honey; you can also add vanilla extract or pureed fruit to enhance the flavor. Rich in fiber and omega-3 fatty acids, this dessert is easy on the stomach and is also high in omega-3 fatty acids.

Try black bean brownies for a baked treat. You can make a dense, fudgy brownie that is high in protein and fiber by blending black beans with cocoa powder, eggs, and a small amount of sugar.

ADVICE FOR EATING DESSERTS MODERATELY AND WITHOUT FEELING GUILTY

Moderation and thoughtful decision-making are key to enjoying desserts guilt-free. Portion control is important; if you want to satisfy your sweet tooth without overloading your system, go for smaller portions rather than indulging in large servings. Using smaller plates or bowls can help you control portion sizes.

Desserts should be balanced with nutrient-dense meals throughout the day to help support overall health and minimize any potential digestive discomfort. If you do plan to have dessert, make sure your other meals are high in vegetables, lean proteins, and healthy fats. You can also avoid overindulging and better control your cravings by spacing out your dessert consumption.

Ultimately, it's critical to pay attention to your body's signals. Observe how different foods affect your symptoms and make adjustments accordingly. If a certain ingredient tends to set off symptoms, look for alternatives or substitutes that suit your needs better.

DESSERT SUBSTITUTES THAT FULFILL CRAVINGS WITHOUT ACTIVATING SIDE EFFECTS

It takes ingenuity and a thorough understanding of your dietary requirements to find dessert substitutes that satiate cravings without aggravating Crohn's disease. A great substitute is frozen yogurt, which is made with lactose-free yogurt and blended fruits; it's a creamy, satisfying treat that's easy on the digestive system, and you can top it with small amounts of nuts or seeds for extra crunch and nutrition.

Another choice is rice pudding, which is a combination of white rice, almond milk, and a small amount of honey. It is a filling dessert that can be eaten warm or cold, is easy on the stomach, and tastes good when flavored with cinnamon or vanilla. Rice pudding is a versatile and calming option for those with Crohn's disease.

Think about creating energy bites with oats, nut butter, and a tiny bit of honey. These easy-to-make, no-bake treats can be personalized with dried fruits or seeds. Energy bites provide a wholesome, portable dessert that's rich in protein and healthy fats, helping to sate sweet cravings without upsetting stomachs.

CHAPTER FIVE

PARTICULAR DIETS AND LIMITATIONS

ADVICE FOR MEETING PARTICULAR NUTRITIONAL REQUIREMENTS

To ensure that your dishes remain safe for those who have gluten intolerance or celiac disease, it's important to understand the substitutions and adjustments that must be made to maintain flavor and nutrition when catering to specific dietary needs like dairy-free or gluten-free diets. When cooking gluten-free, substitute wheat-based products with alternatives like rice flour, almond flour, or gluten-free oats. Many recipes can be modified by using gluten-free pasta, bread, and baking mixes.

If you follow a dairy-free diet, there are many plant-based milk substitutes that you can use in baking and cooking, such as almond, soy, and oat milk. Dairy-free cheese, yogurt, and butter are also easily found in most supermarkets and can help preserve the richness and creaminess of your recipes without making people with lactose intolerance or dairy allergies feel uncomfortable.

Cross-contamination is an important consideration when cooking for people with special dietary needs. To ensure that you consistently meet these dietary needs, always use separate utensils and cooking surfaces to prevent traces of dairy or gluten from contaminating food. Labeling and organizing ingredients in your kitchen can also help.

RECIPES FIT FOR A VEGETARIAN OR VEGAN DIET

It takes knowledge of plant-based proteins and nutrient-dense ingredients to create recipes that work for vegan or vegetarian diets. Legumes, such as lentils, chickpeas, and beans, are great sources of protein for soups, stews, and salads. Tofu and tempeh are flexible options for adding protein to stir-fries, curries, and sandwiches.

Nuts and seeds like almonds, chia seeds, and flaxseeds can be added to meals for an extra boost of healthy fats and proteins.

A variety of vegetables, grains, and nuts can enhance vegetarian diets. Whole grains like quinoa, brown rice, and farro not only add texture and flavor to dishes but also provide essential nutrients.

Experimenting with spices and herbs can also enhance the flavors of your vegan or vegetarian dishes, making them delicious and satisfying. When creating vegan recipes, it's important to take into account the role of animal-derived ingredients and find suitable plant-based alternatives. For example, in baking, replace eggs with flaxseed or chia seed gels. Use nutritional yeast to add a cheesy flavor to dishes.

LOW-RESIDUE FOOD SELECTIONS FOR PERIODS OF OUTBURSTS

Low-residue meals emphasize easily digested, low-fiber foods like white rice, plain pasta, and tender meats like chicken or fish; high-fiber foods like raw vegetables, whole grains, and nuts can aggravate symptoms. During flare-ups, people with Crohn's disease often benefit from low-residue diets, which help reduce the frequency and volume of stools.

Cooked veggies (carrots, potatoes, squash) are easier on the stomach and can be a part of low-residue meals. Fruits (applesauce, canned peaches) that have been peeled and seeded can also be good choices. These foods can be added to soups, stews, and casseroles to make a nourishing and calming meal during flare-ups.

Small, frequent meals rather than large portions can facilitate digestion and help manage symptoms more successfully. Fluids like broths, clear soups, and electrolyte-replenishing drinks are important to include during flare-ups. Herbal teas and diluted juices can also help maintain hydration without irritating the digestive tract.

ADDING ANTI-INFLAMMATORY SUBSTANCES TO YOUR FOODS

By lowering inflammation and improving overall gut health, anti-inflammatory ingredients can help manage

Crohn's disease. Two such powerful anti-inflammatory ingredients are ginger and turmeric, which can be added to teas, smoothies, and stir-fries to help soothe the digestive system. Turmeric, with its active compound curcumin, is an excellent anti-inflammatory that can be added to soups, stews, and curries.

Flaxseed oil and chia seeds can be added to your morning smoothie or used as a main source of protein in your meals. Omega-3 fatty acids are known for their anti-inflammatory qualities; they can be found in fatty fish like salmon and mackerel, as well as flaxseeds and chia seeds. Eating these foods can help reduce inflammation and support heart health.

Antioxidants and anti-inflammatory compounds can be found in leafy green vegetables, like spinach and kale, which can be added to salads, smoothies, and cooked dishes. Nuts, seeds, and berries are also great sources of anti-inflammatory nutrients. Including a range of these foods in your daily diet can help manage symptoms and promote overall health.

ADAPTING RECIPES TO INDIVIDUAL DIETARY RESTRICTIONS AND TASTE PREFERENCES

Meals can be made both fun and safe by modifying recipes to accommodate individual taste preferences and dietary restrictions. To start, find out what special needs your guests may have (allergies, intolerances, personal dislikes, etc.). If someone doesn't like a certain vegetable, you can replace it with one that is similar in texture or nutritional value.

Try experimenting with different seasoning blends to keep meals healthy and in compliance with dietary needs. For people who need to cut back on sugar, think about using natural sweeteners like stevia or monk fruit. For those who follow low-sodium or sugar-free diets, use herbs and spices to enhance flavor without adding extra salt or sugar.

CHAPTER SIX

FAQS & FREQUENTLY ASKED QUESTIONS

HANDLING VARIATIONS IN WEIGHT WITH A CROHN'S DIET

A Crohn's-friendly diet aims to provide adequate nutrition while addressing symptoms that can lead to weight gain or loss. Since Crohn's disease affects digestion and nutrient absorption, managing fluctuations in weight is common. To start, focus on foods that are easier to digest, like cooked vegetables, lean proteins like chicken or fish, and refined grains. These foods are gentler on the digestive system and can help maintain a healthy weight.

Maintaining energy levels and preventing drastic weight fluctuations can also be achieved by eating small, frequent meals throughout the day. Keeping a food diary can help identify trigger foods that may contribute to weight changes, allowing for better management of symptoms over time.

Finally, incorporating calorie-dense foods like nut butter, avocados, and healthy oils to boost caloric intake without exacerbating symptoms.

Maintaining a healthy weight with Crohn's disease requires balancing nutrition and managing symptoms. Consult a registered dietitian to customize your diet to your unique needs and way of life. They can offer individualized advice on how to plan meals, take supplements, and deal with weight fluctuations in a way that promotes overall health and optimal nutrition.

MANAGING NUTRITIONAL LIMITATIONS IN SOCIAL CONTEXTS

It can be difficult to navigate social settings when you have Crohn's disease, but with planning and communication, you can still enjoy social gatherings without sacrificing your health. Before you go to an event, let the host or restaurant staff knows about your dietary restrictions; most will be accommodating and will adjust dishes to your specifications.

You can also offer to bring a dish that fits your diet to make sure you have something to eat.

Eat simple, well-cooked dishes like grilled chicken or fish, steamed vegetables, and rice. If you're dining out, check the menu in advance or give the chef a call to discuss your dietary needs; many restaurants are willing to customize meals to accommodate specific dietary restrictions, including those related to Crohn's disease. The focus should be on foods that are gentle on your digestive system and avoid trigger foods that may exacerbate symptoms.

Socializing can be made more enjoyable and less stressful by keeping a positive attitude and being proactive about your dietary needs. It's important to remember to stay hydrated and pay attention to your body's cues during social events. You can navigate dietary restrictions in social settings with confidence and make sure that your needs are met without feeling alone or deprived if you plan and advocate for your health.

TAKING CARE OF THE COMMON NUTRIENT DEFICIENCIES IN CROHN'S PATIENTS

Because of malabsorption, inflammation, and dietary restrictions, Crohn's disease patients frequently have deficiencies in important nutrients. These include iron, vitamin B12, calcium, vitamin D, and magnesium. It is crucial to monitor and treat these deficiencies with diet and supplementation under the guidance of a healthcare professional or registered dietitian.

Include foods high in iron, such as lean meats, spinach, and fortified cereals, to help prevent anemia, which is a common problem among Crohn's patients. If absorption is compromised, get your vitamin B12 from animal sources, such as fish, poultry, and dairy products, or take supplements. Calcium and vitamin D are important for strong bones; include dairy products that have been fortified with these nutrients, or consult a doctor before taking supplements.

Supplements may be required to maintain optimal nutrient levels, especially during flare-ups or periods of increased disease activity. A balanced diet rich in nutrient-dense foods combined with targeted supplementation can help mitigate the impact of Crohn's disease on nutrient status and overall health. Regular blood tests can help identify deficiencies early, allowing for timely intervention.

SUGGESTIONS FOR EATING OUT WHILE FOLLOWING A CROHN'S DISEASE DIET

To keep symptoms under control and prevent trigger foods, dining out with Crohn's disease requires careful planning. Look for restaurants that have a reputation for providing healthier, customizable options; in particular, look for menu items that include simple starches like rice or potatoes, vegetables, and grilled or steamed proteins, as these are generally easier to digest.

Ask for sauces and dressings on the side to control ingredient amounts and steer clear of potential triggers like spicy or highly seasoned dishes. Choose simple preparations and steer clear of fried or overly processed foods, which can exacerbate symptoms.

When placing an order, make sure the server or chef is aware of your dietary needs.

Plan and advocate for your dietary needs to minimize the impact of Crohn's disease on your health and well-being. Eat less by sharing dishes or managing portion sizes to reduce the risk of overeating.

Stay hydrated with water or herbal teas, avoiding carbonated beverages and alcohol that can irritate the digestive system.

RECOGNIZING SUPPLEMENTS' FUNCTION IN SYMPTOM MANAGEMENT

Because malabsorption and nutrient deficiencies are common in Crohn's patients, supplements can help fill in the gaps in essential vitamins and minerals that may not be adequately absorbed from food alone. Supplements play a crucial role in managing symptoms and supporting overall health for individuals with Crohn's disease.

A balanced diet and medication regimen prescribed by your healthcare team can be supplemented with a variety of supplements, such as probiotics to support gut health, omega-3 fatty acids for anti-inflammatory benefits, and multivitamins to address potential deficiencies. It is important to discuss your supplement regimen with a healthcare provider or registered dietitian to ensure safety and effectiveness.

Selecting supplements from reliable brands and following suggested dosages are important. You should also keep a close eye on how supplements are working for you because everyone's tolerance and absorption are different.

Finally, you should regularly discuss your supplement regimen with medical professionals so that it can be modified in response to evolving symptoms or treatment plans.

For those with Crohn's disease, incorporating supplements into your daily routine can help with symptom management, improve nutritional status, and improve overall quality of life. You can create a customized supplement strategy that meets your needs and supports long-term health and well-being by keeping lines of communication open and working closely with healthcare providers.

www.ingramcontent.com/pod-product-compliance
Lightning Source LLC
Chambersburg PA
CBHW071840210526
45479CB00001B/217